Health Care Information Technology

The Hardware and Software Focus:

Critical Factors for EMR Implementation

2nd Edition

ISBN-10 0615447775

ISBN-13 9780615447773

Printed in the United States of America

First Printing, 2011

1

For permission requests and ordering information: write to the publisher, addressed "Attention: Book Coordinator," at the address below.

HCITSC LLC
P.O. Box 3388
Federal Way, WA 98063

How to Use This Book

Attention Health Care and Healthcare Information Technology Industry: Regardless of what stage you are in with your organization's EMR, revenue cycle, payment processing, and/or medical implementation, you can benefit from this book. What you are about to read is an attempt to demystify common sources of confusion and shed light on solutions to typical problems.

Health Care Information Technology is an exciting and valuable new field, it is important to understand the requirements necessary to ensure that the software and hardware used within the industry support the goals of hospitals and small providers around the nation. Today, legislation such as the American Recovery and Reinvestment Act of 2009 (ARRA), the Health Insurance Portability and Accountability Act of 1996 (HIPAA), and the Health Information Technology for Economic and Clinical Health (HITECH) Act continue to add additional requirements to medical IT systems.

This book is intended to accomplish all of the following goals:

•Clear up essential misunderstandings related to terminology
•Show readers the extent of the problems that affect the field today
•Summarize key legislation that affects the industry
•Provide readers with a pathway to entering Health Care IT
•Introduce the Health Care Information Technology Service Center

•Give readers a handy guide of industry definitions

Reasons for 2nd Revision 2011

The author and HC-IT-SC want to begin by apologizing to those who purchased the first edition. This revised edition corrects and improves upon that volume by offering a more positive message to those in the health care industry. It is intended to serve as a reference guide for all, presenting a constructive perspective on the health care industry and its many components. Creating and adding to this book should be a community effort. Please feel free to provide request to add information within the book.

Endorsements of the book include:
Healthcare Information Technology Association
Healthcare Information Technology Stimulus Center

Proofreaders and reviewers of this book include:
Laura Brenner, PhD; Laura Brenner Writing Services

About the Book

This book has been created to address the implications and ramifications of several important pieces of legislation: namely, the American Recovery and Reinvestment Act of 2009 (ARRA), the Health Insurance Portability and Accountability Act of 1996 (HIPAA), and the Health Information Technology for Economic and Clinical Health (HITECH) Act. This book provides the reader with key research and information from both scholarly and industry sources. In the author's opinion, this information is critical if those working in the health care IT industry wish to make quality decisions. All courses, terms, degrees, procedures, recommendations, and certifications within this book and/or associated with HC-IT-SC have been trademarked and copyrighted. There is a penalty for attempting to recreate this information.

Information for Suggested Sales Leads

Independent Book Stores
Health Care Organizations
Hospital Book Stores
Colleges
Book Stores

Contents

Introduction

Health Care Information Technology (HCIT) is a unique field that continues to evolve. It consists of many components, has its own specific terminology, is a part of many different fields, and brings together many organizations through the use of various information systems. Perhaps most notably, HCIT extends to various types of medical applications.

Currently, the field suffers from serious problems that need to be addressed immediately. The Health Care Information Technology Stimulus Center (hereafter, HC-IT-SC) was created to assist the Health Care Information Technology field by focusing on the software and hardware it utilizes.

Some of the different types of organizations that use Health Care Information Systems consist of hospitals, urgent care centers, insurance companies, and private doctor's offices. With this in mind, Information Technology (or IT) within the field of health care consists of software and hardware components that follow the platforms of the networking development life cycle of medical applications, other software, and other hardware components.

On the next page is a chart showing the *Top-Down Model and Network Development Life Cycle* for the world of Health Care Information Technology.[1]

---

[1]   "Computer Networks," 2002

THE TOP-DOWN MODEL AND NETWORK DEVELOPMENT LIFE CYCLE FOR HEALTH CARE INFORMATION TECHNOLOGY	
Top-Down Model	**Information Systems Development Process**
Business	Strategic business planning Business processing
Applications	Systems development life cycle Systems analysis and design Application development life cycle
Data	Database analysis and design Database distribution analysis
Network	Network development life cycle Network analysis and design
Technology	Physical network design Network implementation Technology analysis

One should note that this chart presents an *ideal* description of the way that an IT system should be designed and implemented within the health care industry. In other words, developers and IT professionals first examine the field from a bird's eye view before determining specific applications and implementation that will solve a particular problem or improve workflow.

Unfortunately, this does not describe the way that IT has been developed and implemented thus far.

Rather than follow the "Top-Down" model outlined above, the health care industry has made the mistake of taking a "Bottom-Up" approach to IT—that is to say, software and hardware have been developed without an ultimate regard for where they will be implemented, how they will integrate with existing systems or networks, and what the costs and timelines of implementation will be.

As a result, hospitals across the United States have been left with a number of problems and logistical nightmares as a result of rushed or ill-conceived implementation that most certainly did *not* follow the top-down model. As of the time of this book's publication, a number of health care organizations have had difficulty over the last year collecting payments electronically as a result of IT issues. This lack of foresight and planning has directly translated into an industry-wide loss of several billion dollars.

The field of Health Care Information Technology (HCIT) is progressing very fast as it attempts to address these and other issues. While this brings new awareness to the value of the field, it also creates a number of terminology mix-ups with other similar fields. Because of the unique lexicon of HCIT, one can quickly become overwhelmed with a new vocabulary and feel lost when attempting to decipher field-specific documents and other communications.

In addition, Health Care Information Technology is faced with serious problems regarding miscommunication, a general lack of understanding regarding the field, and unclear definitions in terms of how computer hardware and software facilitate information transfer within the field.

This book was created to help solve the issues related to terminology and communication that exist in the Health Care Information Technology field. Furthermore, it demonstrates how our organization, the Healthcare Information Technology Stimulus Center (HC-IT-SC), can provide solutions.

Here are some critical acronyms used within the industry. The following list includes definitions and when/how each term should be properly used.

- Health Information Management, when used in this field, should refer to HIM, HIT, RHIA, CHIA, Health (care) Information Management.

- Healthcare Information Technology, the hardware and software focus, when used in this field, should refer to Healthcare IT.
- IT, when used in this field, should refer to HC-IT, HCIT, and Healthcare Information Technology, Health Care Information Technology.
- Healthcare Informatics, when used in this field, should refer to Medical Applications and Medical Software.
- Health Information Administration, when used in this field, should refer to office and administrative procedures of all health care practices.
- Health Information Management, Healthcare Information Technology software and hardware, Health Informatics, and Health Administration, when used in this field, should refer to Health Information Systems toolkit (Healthcare Information Technology and/or Health Information Management techniques and scopes).

Terminology Defined

Health Care Information Technology vs. Health Information Management

Two terms that often get mixed up are "Health Care Information Technology" and "Health Information Management."

Health Care Information Technology is the application of information processing—which involves both computer hardware and software—to store, retrieve, and share health care information. Health Care Information Technology allows for data and knowledge within the industry to be communicated to a number of agents, which greatly aids the decision-making process. HCIT also involves networking and building computer and communication systems to transmit this health care information. Likewise, Health Care Information Technology involves the engineering of new information systems.[2]

Health Care Information Technology's minimum components include a server to store data, a client computer with an operating system installed, and software that addresses each organization's unique needs. Most components of a medical application are installed and configured depending on the type of data that will be transmitted to and from it.

Health Information Management, on the other hand, is the practice of maintenance and care of health records by traditional and electronic means in hospitals, physician's office clinics, health departments, health insurance companies, and other facilities that provide health care or maintenance of health records. Health informatics and health care information technology are utilized in Health Information Management.[3]

---

[2]   "Health Information Technology," 2010
[3]   "Article Search Results for Medical Cash Applications Specialist," 2010

Health Information Management also includes gathering data, analyzing it, and making it available to those who need it. Its ultimate objective is to enable the delivery of quality health care to the public.

EMR vs. EHR

EMR (Electronic Medical Record) and EHR (Electronic Health Record) are two terms that are often used interchangeably in this and other resources. They are interrelated, but there are a few distinctions between the two terms.

In his medical blog, Houston Neal, Marketing Director at Software Advice, clearly outlined the differences between EHR and EMR; he used the definitions recently drafted by National Alliance for Health Information Technology (NAHIT). According to NAHIT's definitions, an **EMR** is "the electronic record of health-related information on an individual that is created, gathered, managed, and utilized by licensed clinicians and staff from *a single organization* that is involved in the individual's health and care."

An **EHR** (Electronic Health Record) is "the collective electronic record of health-related information on an individual that is created and gathered cumulatively across *more than one* health care organization and is managed and consulted by licensed clinicians and staff involved in the individual's health and care."[4]

In more practical terms, an individual's record from a single organization is an EMR; an individual's record pieced together from more than one health care organization is an EHR. Under this definition, because a single provider may create an EMR only through its hardware and software systems, EMR is used more commonly and where appropriate.

In countries like India, there are various disparities with regard to access to health care between urban and rural regions, poor health

---

[4]   Neal, 2010

indicators, raising burden of communicable and non-communicable diseases, and geographical barriers for the delivery of health services particularly in north and northeastern states. In addition, disasters such as earthquakes, famine, floods, epidemics of diseases, etc., generate the need of public health systems that can adequately address community health problems.

Public health informatics discipline in India is still in the nascent stage. The introduction of telemedicine in the year 2000 by one of the major hospital firms, Apollo's Project in Andhra Pradesh, had led to a steady growth in deployment of ICTs in the region primarily focused on health care services, e.g., Tele-cardiology, Tele-ophthalmology, Tele-oncology, Electronic Medical Records (EMRs), Hospital Management Information Systems, etc.

Data and Medical Applications

Health Information Management manages different types of patient data.

Data is defined as various types of information, usually formatted in a specific way.

In the Health Care Field, the data used includes the Patient's Information (that is, *Name, Address, Social Security Number, and Medical Insurance Information*), and the Patient's ID Number (defined as the *MRN, or Medical Record Number*).

In the Health Care Information Technology field, the protection of data is done through the use of *Usernames, Passwords, MRN, and Policies and Procedures.*

Let us first define these previous terms for better clarity.

Usernames and Passwords are unique sets of characters for the use of one specific person.

The National Committee on Vital and Health Statistics (NCVHS) defines an <u>MRN</u> (Medical Record Number) as a process of identifying a patient. It further explains that each provider organization keeps and maintains a Master Patient Index (MPI), and the MRN is issued and maintained through this index.

The MRN, according to NCVHS, is also used to identify an individual and his or her medical record/information. The numbering system—plus the content and format of the MRN—is mostly specific to the individual organization.[5]

The <u>Policies and Procedures</u> vary from organization to organization, depending on that organization's needs. For example, HIPAA is a policy that all health care organizations have to follow. HIPAA now has standards and guidelines that must be met when dealing with Health Care Information Technology.

For example, the act sets certain guidelines with regard to health care computer security, due to the fact that systems and/or applications may vary widely in how actively and how they prevent unauthorized users from accessing data.

Medical Applications are defined as unique applications installed on a client computer that have proven to be in compliance with all policies and procedures.

Additionally, a medical application is any computer program that is used within a health care organization. For example, it can include software that connects to medical devices, hearing aids, medical imaging systems, remote patient monitoring and diagnostics, or medical alarm applications.

---

[5]   "Existing Medical Record Number (MRN) based identification," 2010

The History of Computers

It is amazing how computers evolved from using our own fingers and toes to count to the complex technology that the world has now. The oldest clue to the earliest form of a computer was the carvings of prime numbers into a bone, found sometime around 8500 BCE (Before the Common Era).

Sometime between 1000 BCE and 500 BCE, the abacus evolved. This instrument had movable beads whose positions changed in such a way that its user could enter numbers and perform mathematical computations.

But the world's first mechanical calculator was created by Leonardo da Vinci in 1500. Then in 1642, Blaise Pascal's adding machine replaced Leonardo's basic calculator, moving computing forward again.

During the 19th century, English mathematician Charles Babbage introduced plans for a machine called the Babbage Difference Engine. Though it was designed to calculate numbers, it was able to print mathematical tables. Since Babbage was unable to construct the actual device, he received significant criticism. This challenged Babbage to address the limitations of his design. So he next developed plans for the Babbage Analytical Engine. This computing device would use punch cards as the control mechanism for calculations, a feature that would allow previously performed calculations to be used for future ones.

Soon Babbage met Ada Byron Lovelace, a woman who was passionate about mathematics. Lovelace saw new possibilities for the Analytical Machine, including the production of graphics and music. His project became a reality with her help. She documented how the device would calculate Bernoulli numbers. Lovelace subsequently was recognized for writing the world's first computer program. A computer language was even named after her by the U.S. Department of Defense in 1979.

Every computer that was developed built on the successes of previous ones. The first programmable computer arrived in 1943 named the

Turing COLOSSUS. It was developed to decode German messages during World War II.

In 1946, ENIAC (Electronic Numerical Integrator And Computer), "The Giant Brain," became the first electronic digital computer developed by the U.S. Army during World War II.

Then in 1951, the U.S. Census Bureau became the first government agency to buy the first commercial computer built in the United States—the UNIVAC (Universal Automatic Computer).

Soon people began connecting computers together, point-to-point, allowing them to communicate. This type of communication evolved into more and more complex capabilities that ultimately resulted in the creation of the original Internet in the late 1960s and early 1970s.

In 1977, computers were expanded to consumers with the release of the Apple computer. Soon after in 1981, the IBM Personal Computer (PC) for consumers was released even though IBM mainframes were already in use by government and corporations at that time.

The main protocol used to run the modern Internet, TCP/IP (Transmission Control Protocol/Internet Protocol), was created in the 1970s by the U.S. Department of Defense. Meanwhile in 1980, Tim Berners-Lee developed the World Wide Web and CERN (the European Organization for Nuclear Research) released the first web server in 1991. The development of the web was the fundamental technology that popularized the Internet around the world.

Current computer technologies include word processing, games, email, maps, medical systems, data manipulation, and streaming data. Computers continue to evolve at a breakneck pace.[6]

---

[6] "The History of the Computer," 2010

Computers and Health Care Information Technology

As we have previously discussed, HCIT is the computer technology—consisting of both hardware and software—that is used within health care organizations.

The first computers intended for business use arrived on the market in the 1960s, and they replaced both the low-cost/low-performance drum memory devices and the high-cost/high-performance systems that used vacuum tubes (and later transistors) as memory.

Computer hardware and software started being used in wider numbers around 1975, when the first home computer, the Altair 8800, became popular. Though the term "medical application" was not yet in use, software and hardware components were already being used in the radiology field.

On November 8, 1895, Wilhelm Conrad Röntgen accidentally produced an image cast from his cathode ray generator (an X-ray). This may have been the beginning of the discovery of the first medical applications, which would have consisted of computer hardware and images, but lacked coding.

The medical applications, computer software, and computer hardware in HCIT have evolved over the years and include the advancement of medical devices, hearing aids, medical imaging systems, remote patient monitoring and diagnostics, and medical alarm applications.

A suggested *workable* set of requirements for a medical application are as follows: First, that the application be paired with a medical device, hearing aid, medical imaging system (or remote patient monitoring and diagnostics and medical alarm applications), and second, that the top-down development life cycle is used to create the application's software.

Some medical applications use proprietary software; this depends on the organization's needs. Some medical applications are created by a software developer for a single organization.

American Recovery and Reinvestment Act Meaning and Use

The American Recovery and Reinvestment Act of 2009 (ARRA) was signed into law by President Obama on February 17, 2009. In this bill, $59 billion was allocated for health care with approximately $20 billion designated for EMR adoption. Obviously, many doctors who are interested in EMR want to know how they can claim some part of this massive $20 billion allocation.

A total of $17 billion will be distributed as incentives paid out in the form of increased Medicare and Medicaid payments. Incentives will start in 2011 and be paid over five years for a physician who can show "meaningful use" of an EMR system (what constitutes meaningful use is to be defined later in "Legislation"). Conversely, physicians who do not prove "meaningful use" will be reprimanded via lower Medicare payments. Hospital physicians will not be affected.

Those entitled to some portion of the stimulus money will also have to use a "certified" EHR system. As with the term "meaningful use," the definition of a "certified" system has not been defined by the government.

The maximum a provider can receive is $44,000 over a period of five years, paid either in a lump sum or through payments determined by HHS. Furthermore, in order to be eligible for these funds, the physician must also use electronic prescribing in a meaningful way.

Health Care Information Technology Policy and Standards Committee Better Known as the Health Information Technology Policy

While the details of "meaningful use" under ARRA are in need of clarification, the act does require that in order for payments to be made, a physician must demonstrate that the EHR technology provides for the electronic exchange of health information to improve the quality of health care activities, such as promoting care coordination. He or she must also submit information on clinical quality measures as specified by HHS.

Under the provisions of ARRA, a Health Information Policy Committee will focus on development of a nationwide health information infrastructure; in pursuit of this goal, the Committee will recommend standards, implementation specifications, and certification criteria.

It is clear that the timeline for implementing electronic health records to receive federal incentive payments will create demand for a variety of qualified professional services between now and 2012.

With respect to this book and to clarify the mix up for the purpose of a clear understanding the above policy should have been named the "Health Information Management" policy with the true definitions in mind.

Summary of ARRA Details for HCIT Implementation

- Provision of $40,000 in incentives (beginning in 2011) for physicians to use EHRs
- Provision of funds to states to coordinate and promote interoperable EHRs

- Acceleration of the construction of the National Health Information Network (NHIN)
- Creation of grant and loan programs
- Development of educational programs to train clinicians in EHR use and increase the number of health care IT professionals
- Creation of extension programs to facilitate regional adoption efforts

How and Why HC-IT-SC can help

The EMR/Health Care Information Technology field is a very private industry that demands a high level of understanding before new organizations can begin to take advantage of its opportunities.

HC-IT-SC can help your organization (1) prepare for the demands of the EMR/Health Care Information Technology field and/or (2) assist other organizations.

HC-IT-SC has done extensive research and has direct access to a number of industry professionals.

We are "Industry Certified" professionals.
As such, our certification and experience provides your organization with the following benefits:
- Training
  - We train company staff.
  - We focus on Hardware/Software requirements of the EMR and HIPAA stimulus package.
- Representation
  - After training, we can represent the stimulus package for certified companies.
- Implementation
  - We create a roadmap to a successful EMR implementation.

HC-IT-SC and ITC

The Health Care Information Technology Stimulus Center and Information Technology Center were created and implemented to assist health care providers access the $20 billion of recent federal funds created through the American Recovery and Reinvestment Act of 2009. The act's goals are stated as follows:

> *Lower Healthcare Costs by Investing in Electronic Information Technology Systems: Use health information technology to lower the cost of health care. Invest $20 billion a year over the next five years to move the U.S. health care system to broad adoption of standards-based electronic health information systems, including electronic health records (from the Washington Post).*

Naturally, the $20 billion federal investment has opened the door for new jobs. However, the training for these new positions was not available until the Information Technology Center launched in 2009.

Problems with the Industry

As previously mentioned, the Health Care Information Technology field is currently facing serious problems with regard to miscommunication, a lack of understanding, and a lack of definition in where computer hardware and software fit within the context of all the data being transmitted in the field. Furthermore, Health Care Information Technology is facing a possible problem with the HITECH legislation, specifically with regard to how HHS will interpret what a certified EMR is.

Faced with these challenges, HC-IT-SC and its research team will conduct detailed research on Health Care Information Technology, cell phones, and various medical applications, as well as how these different parts interact within a larger program. Emphasis will be placed in the research on the processes and technologies involved in creating, managing, visualizing, and understanding a diverse array of digital content, as well as how this content affects individuals, groups, organizations, societies, and globally distributed systems.

Another issue to consider is that any data is only part of a "knowledge life cycle" that progresses from (1) data to (2) knowledge to (3) research. Thus, to incorporate new technologies, support new classes of applications and services, and meet new requirements and challenges, new players in this field will need to scale and adapt their efforts to account for unforeseen events and uncertainties across multiple dimensions. These dimensions include types of applications, network size and topology, mobility patterns, heterogeneity of devices, and networking technologies.

Implementation and Compliance

Successful implementation within one's organization should include a team of professionals from the fields of IT service management, IT compliance, software change management, deployment and release management, and IT portfolio management. HC-IT-SC's solutions ensure that your requests, changes, and releases are consistently captured, viewed, and tracked across your entire IT organization, including service desk, application development, and network operations. Furthermore, through defining and managing processes, HC-IT-SC's service, change, and release management solutions can help you easily achieve IT compliance.

Compliance Factors

One thing that health care organizations should realize is that compliance is mandatory. However, the *manner* of compliance is more crucial than a mere pass-or-fail of the HIPAA guidelines.

How compliance is achieved will determine an organization's ability to bill, collect, and input data. In certain cases, it may even affect an organization's financial and operational performance.

The following are guidelines that will help in successful implementation and compliance:

Awareness of Rules
There is a tremendous amount of misinformation and misunderstanding about the terminology, definitions, policies, transactions, and rules that govern the Health Care Information Technology field. Thus, awareness of federal, state, and company-level rules is very important for successful implementation and legal compliance. In addition to seeking advice from consultants, we suggest that you read and follow any applicable sets of rules.

Change Leadership and Business Process Reengineering
There will always be resistance to change if it is viewed as a disruption to the customary way of doing things. However, if change is viewed as an expansion or advancement, it will be welcomed and even embraced. View compliance and implementation in the context of Change Leadership and Business Process Reengineering.

A Need for Urgency
There is an urgent need to comply and implement *now*. The more an organization delays, the more the task will seem monumental to those charged with implementation.

Evaluation of all Systems and Processes
Health care organizations conduct gap analysis to develop a roadmap in making decisions regarding remediating, upgrading, replacing, or outsourcing systems and processes. Since the cost of remediating legacy systems may be prohibitive for some health care organizations, replacement of noncompliant systems could be a key to assuring compliance and business continuity.

Selection of Systems
To reduce implementation time, the number of interfaces, risk, and total cost of ownership (TCO), the strategy for health care organizations should be focused on selecting systems that provide interoperability

and complete integration.

Evaluation of EMR Implementation Options
The use of an EMR system is particularly important for hospitals to obtain the full benefits of automated clinical documentation. The adoption of EMRs is a drastic operational change, especially for physicians. It can take anywhere from three to nine months on average for clinicians to adapt and recover from the loss of productivity that normally accompanies EMR implementation. If the EMR is not carefully selected and properly implemented, lost physician productivity (25 percent to 40 percent on average) may never be recovered.

Obtaining the Right Tools
It is beneficial to talk with software vendors and learn who they are partnered with in order to implement coding and auto-coding. With the complexity and number of codes, manual coding is not realistic in most cases.

Value of Training
Training is consistently cited as a top critical success factor, and the number of staff members who need training is normally underestimated. The level of training needed within an organization will vary, but it is absolutely vital to provide training to key members at all levels.

Successful Implementation with HC-IT-SC

As previously mentioned, it is HC-IT-SC's purpose to bridge the communication gap that invariably results from a number of differences in terminologies. We also act as a resource center to document and regulate Health Care Information Technology, focusing on software and hardware.

We are "industry certified" professionals who offer training, representation, and implementation. As industry certified professionals with extensive experience in the field, we understand the importance of establishing a compliance structure that is clear, effective, and consistent with business objectives.

HC-IT-SC can provide you with expert services to ensure successful implementation, compliance, and project completion.

Medical Applications in Health Care Information Technology

There are various medical applications that can be used within your health care organization. However, your stimulus team needs to evaluate your organization's needs first and ensure that security is kept as a primary goal throughout any implementation of Health Care Information Technology. Your applications should not run the risk of access by hackers or other competing organizations.

To comply with HIPAA, you should include a confidentiality agreement during the implementation stage of your proprietary systems. This can simply be a part of your EMR stipulations.

Below is a sample agreement:

The Collaboratee agrees to keep all of the Collaborator's business secrets confidential at all times. Collaborator's business secrets include any information regarding the Collaborator's customers, supplies, finances, research, development, manufacturing processes, or any other technical or business information.

The Collaboratee agrees not to make any unauthorized copies of any of the Collaborator's business secrets or information without Collaborator's consent, nor to remove any of Collaborator's business secrets or information from the Collaborator facilities.

WHEREAS, "Collaborator" wishes to assure that the confidential and proprietary information is protected from disclosure and only used by the Collaboratee for the purpose of evaluating and/or creating, developing, designing or accepting a Collaboration Project.

For this business purpose the Collaboratee shall not use any ideas, information, Health Care certifications, employees, classes, companies, business, documents, contacts, computer software programs, corporate operations procedures, marketing plans and methods, customer lists, prospective clients lists (regardless of whether such lists have been distilled or tailored for the specific use of the Disclosing Party), for its sole purpose. In addition, Collaboratee agrees that all information relative to carriers and any of the companies that are the primary source for the Products of "Collaborator" are confidential and are not to be used by Collaboratee, unless Collaboratee has been given permission in writing by "Collaborator" to offer the products, only for joint purpose of this business relationship. This includes all information disclosed in oral, written, graphic, photographic, recorded, diagrammed, digital, electronic or any other form by one party to the other as well as the content of this Agreement and the content of any and all discussions between the parties related to this Agreement or otherwise;

WHEREAS, "Collaborator" wishes to assure that upon completion of the review of the potential business relationship or termination of discussions between the parties, and/or termination of creating or developing permitted Business Purpose, and designing the "Collaborator's" Collaboration Project, that the confidential and proprietary information is returned to the "Collaborator" and/or not disclosed, or used for any purpose, at any time, by the Collaboratee. For the purpose of this Business agreement and Business to Business relationship, all work performed, done, completed, requested to be completed, created, and any and all other works copyrights, exclusive rights, related rights, neighboring rights, works subject to copyright, exclusive rights granted by copyright, moral rights, right to be credited for the work, and Copyright as property right is/are owned wholly, legally, solely, rights of, and created by (your company name).

Collaboratee to this agreement agrees not to compete, either directly or indirectly, with the business ideas, supplies, finances, research, development, manufacturing processes, or any other technical or business information of the (your company name) and affiliates.

The Collaboratee agrees that "not to compete" means not to engage in any manner in a business or activity similar to the business ideas, supplies, finances, research, development, manufacturing processes, or any other technical or business information of the (your company) and affiliates.

The Collaboration term is defined for the purpose of this agreement as - Project thoughts and communication. There are no payment terms attached to this agreement. Agreement states stipulated as contractor in the contractor application agreement. Please see attached.

If this agreement is violated, the (your company name) and affiliates will be entitled to an injunction to prevent such competition, without the need for the buyer to post any bond. In addition, the (your company name) and affiliates will be entitled to any other legal relief.

Stimulus Team

The American Recovery and Reinvestment Act of 2009 has stated within its stipulations that each organization should have an "EMR and HIPAA Economic Stimulus team." An organization's stimulus team should consist of a trainer with a strong educational background and more than 10 years worth of training/teaching experience in an adult environment, specifically in the high-technology arena.

Likewise, the team should contain individuals who hold current certifications and at least a bachelor's degree in Information Technology. The team should have organizational and technical training experience that allows them to prove their ability to identify problems, analyze possible solutions, and determine the best course of action—all of which ensure that your organization's objectives will be successfully met.

This is where HC-IT-SC provides an invaluable benefit to the field. Health Care and Information Technology employees who successfully complete our new certificate program will gain access to many opportunities through certificate program affiliates, allowing them to apply for a greater variety of job opportunities.

Additional criteria for your organization's stimulus team include:
- Demonstration of ability as an effective trainer to deliver clear, concise, and engaging technology training for group and individual audiences
- Use of Internet-focused job search and professional networking techniques
- Demonstration of skills to utilize feedback and make quality improvements in workshop delivery and content
- Demonstration of ability to create and comply with a project plan, timeline, and budget
- Demonstration of ability to collect, input, and report data to maintain records
- Demonstration of familiarity working with hardware and a variety of secure networks across several agencies and locations
- Ability to function effectively both as an independent trainer and as an integrated team member
- Demonstration of ability to recruit and market training workshops, customize standardized, pre-approved brochures and formats, etc.
- Ability to solve problems creatively and effectively.

Training for the Health Care Information Technology field has until now been a major challenge as it has been difficult to find properly trained professionals. Since the ARRA was implemented, many employers have been attempting to hire for these positions. However, many employers are struggling with finding and understanding the key qualifications of job applicants in relation to their needs.

The Information Technology Center has created a program (described below in greater detail) to assist health care organizations in hiring qualified professionals.

In today's rapidly expanding Health Care Information Technology field, aspiring health care and information technology workers will require training, retraining, and skills upgrades to succeed in the Health Care Information Technology workplace. The Information Technology Center has developed the HC-IT Short Certificate program to provide students with the information technology skills that are most useful to the health care industry. This Short Certificate program builds on current IT and Health Care Information Technology industry training.

HC-IT-SC — *Mission, Customers, Purpose, and Services*

HC-IT-SC is a one-stop shop for customers, providing detailed research in one website. HC-IT-SC is the best online resource available for information on Health Care Information Technology. (We invite you to find us online at www.hc-it-sc.com).

HC-IT-SC's customers include health care organizations, health care professionals, and educational organizations that specialize in the field of Health Care Information Technology. Our purpose is to provide fast and reliable technical assistance to our valued customers.

HC-IT-SC's mission is to provide the health care community with tools that can assist with many areas of an organization's health care needs. HC-IT-SC also assists industry members in connecting with EMR professionals—both job seekers and employers.

Our web site is devoted to meeting the changing needs of the Health Care Information Technology industry created by the stipulations of HIPAA and ARRA. It is a leading online resource.

HC-IT-SC and ITC — *Mission, Services, Partners*

HC-IT-SC and the Information Technology Center thrive on assisting the rapidly growing field of Information Technology in the health care sector. We offer training in new technologies to assist people with upgrading their skills for employment. HC-IT-SC and Information Technology Center employees have strong industry-specific backgrounds, which often include several years of experience working with companies such as Microsoft, Group Health, Ohio State University Medical Center, and North Seattle Community College on various IT and health care training projects.

HC-IT-SC and the Information Technology Center's mission is to provide clients with a wealth of information to assist in their professional needs. Furthermore, the ITC trains individuals with the skills needed to fill positions in today's job market.

The Information Technology Center and HC-IT-SC's industry partners include:
- Certified trainers
- Various employment firms

The HC-IT-SC and Information Technology Center can also be used as a tool for:
- Career enhancement and business development
- Displaced workers
- Education and training
- Individuals with disabilities
- Job seekers, hiring managers, and employers.

The Job Training Focus at HC-IT-SC and Information Technology Center includes job titles such as:

- Application Support
- Clinical Systems Support
- Customer Service Representative
- Information Technology Sales
- Instructor
- Medical Customer Service Support
- Medical Help Desk Support
- Medical Record Technician
- Medical Sales
- Office Clerk
- Patient Coordinator
- Radiology Medical Customer Service Support
- Radiology Medical Help Desk Support
- Radiology Systems Support
- Scheduler
- Healthcare Information Technician
- Trainer
- Unit Coordinator

The benefits of the Information Technology Center's new HC-IT Certificate Program include:

- Industry certifications
- Acquiring the capability to be multi-skilled for employment in as many as five different industries
- Updated skills

Information Technology Training Programs

Our training programs are taught by certified professionals. The growing demand for IT jobs and computer-related skills make it a great time to learn new skills or upgrade existing ones. All courses have a five-day training extension for qualified applicants. This is by agency request only.

Our training consists of two major programs: the Certification Program and the Professional Training Program. Below is a detailed breakdown of these programs:

Certification Program
- Healthcare Information Technician Certification
- HC-IT Application Specialist Certification
- HC-IT Implementation Specialist Certification
- Certified PACS Associate Specialist (CPAS)
- Certified PACS Interface Analyst (CPIA)
- Certified PACS System Analyst (CPSA)
- Certified PACS System Manager (CPSM)

Professional Training Program
- Professional Training
- Basic Computer Skills
- Customer Service
- Transitional Skills
- "EMR" Transitional Skills
- Cell/Mobile Phone Technician
- Microsoft Office 2007
- Microsoft Office 2003
- Resume Writing
- Computer Skills
- Health Care and Computers
- Software Testing

31

- New Software in the Workplace
- Front Office Skills

The program also features a job network package option, which provides the successful student with a computer, cell phone, two professional resumes, a professional email account, and two networking contacts to assist with job leads at the time of program completion. (Note: This option requires additional fees.)

Program Development

The Short Certificate will demonstrate to a potential employer your understanding of:
- Customer service
- Digital health care environment
- Information technology
- Medical records
- Medical software systems
- Patient care
- Project management

Implementation
HC-IT Short Certificate program courses are taught in the Information Technology Center's lab, which features tablet notebook PCs, medical software (such as home health software applications), software, and other standard office software programs.

Program Scope
This is an important step in a three-part career and certification pathway in both the health care and IT fields that allows students to obtain four or five industry certifications. This program is intended for currently employed health care professionals, prospective employees, unemployed individuals, licensed practical nurses, pharmacy tech or medical assistants, and individuals with prior IT and/or health care backgrounds.

HC-IT Courses

HC-IT courses are courses in which an Information Technology worker learns to support and/or manage the hardware and software pieces of a health care facility's medical applications.

Certification Programs

Healthcare Information Technician Certification
This certification assists nurses and other medical staff in becoming a super user in their field and/or position. The course curriculum will provide students with an understanding of how to troubleshoot software and hardware used as part of the field of Health Care Information Technology and as part of an organization's Medical Applications.

HC-IT Application Specialist Certification
This certification demonstrates an individual's knowledge of HC-IT medical application skills. This certification is achieved by studying the HC-IT objectives and passing one exam.

HC-IT Implementation Specialist Certification
This certification demonstrates an individual's knowledge of HC-IT medical application implementation skills. It is achieved by studying the HC-IT objectives and passing one exam. The course curriculum includes some computer systems troubleshooting, HIPAA training, computer network troubleshooting skills, and UNIX troubleshooting skills.

Certified PACS Associate Specialist (CPAS)
CPAS certification is achieved by passing two exams: the CPAS-Technical exam (wherein individuals demonstrate their knowledge of general technical skills) and the CPAS-Clinical exam (wherein individuals demonstrate their knowledge of general clinical skills).

Certified PACS Interface Analyst (CPIA)

Individuals who obtain this certification are able to demonstrate their knowledge of DICOM/HL7, including troubleshooting. The course curriculum includes some computer systems troubleshooting, HIPAA training, computer network troubleshooting, and UNIX system troubleshooting.

Certified PACS System Analyst (CPSA)

Individuals who obtain this certification are able to demonstrate their knowledge of PACS components and system administration. The course curriculum includes some computer systems troubleshooting, HIPAA training, computer network troubleshooting, and UNIX system troubleshooting.

Certified PACS System Manager (CPSM)

This is the "capstone" certification. The candidate will be both CPIA and CPSA certified at the time the exam is taken, and in addition, must have advanced and detailed knowledge about subjects such as image quality, security, IHE, and advanced standards development (both DICOM and HL7). The course curriculum includes some computer systems troubleshooting, HIPAA training, computer network troubleshooting, and UNIX system troubleshooting.

Certifications Overview

This unique health care IT career pathway certification provides training for displaced/dissatisfied workers and/or new students to be employed in entry-level positions such as Healthcare Help Desk Technician, Clinical Support Staff, and other call center positions within the HC-IT field.

One must prove to be proficient with respect to both clinical and technical job requirements before obtaining the HC-IT Application Specialist Certification and/or the HC-IT Implementation Specialist Certification.

The following are the prerequisites for the HC-IT Certifications:

- Degree from an accredited college within the last 10 years
- Three years in a health care and/or computer information technology field
- Certification
- Medical certification or licensure of any kind

Scope and Description of HC-IT Courses

HC-IT 201: IT for Healthcare Language

- Understanding of HCPC and codes, and HIPAA and CPT codes
- Understanding of the different types of workflow processes in the health care setting
- Understanding of the health care processes

HC-IT 202: Introduction to the IT for Healthcare

- Environment and technology
- Understanding of the health care policies in the workplace
- Exposure to health care staff process
- Health care software and hardware vendors

HC-IT 203: Mobile Devices in the Healthcare Environment

- Understanding smartphones, PDAs, medical modalities, laptops, and desktops in a health care setting

HC-IT 204: Business Processes in the Healthcare Environment

- The history of health care, health care facilities, information technology in a health care setting
- The differences between HC-IT, HIM, and informatics in a health care setting

HC-IT 205: Successful Medical Implementations

- Important factors of implementation including: management involvement, development, risk of implementation, trial implementation, and additional critical factors within the organization

HC-IT 206: Financial Workflow in the Healthcare Environment

- Information on the clinical data repository, nursing and physician (and other caregiver) documentation systems, clinical decision support system, results reporting system, electronic medication administration system, and pharmacy system

Certification Training and Exams

HC-IT-SC's Certification Training has the following suggested prerequisites:

- Health care or information technology background
- Two- or four-year degree
- Willingness to travel for employment
- Ability to pass a background check

The HC-IT Application Specialist Certification and/or HC-IT Implementation Specialist Certification exams each consists of at least 50 multiple-choice questions and have a 30-minute time limit. All exams require a minimum score of 70 percent in order to pass. If the candidate does not pass, he or she must purchase a second approval to try again, but may only take the exam a maximum of three times within twelve months, which requires the purchase of three separate approval codes. The exam questions will be selected randomly from a pool of questions, ensuring that multiple exam attempts will ask the candidate questions they have not previously encountered.

Detailed Course Training Descriptions

Healthcare Information Technician Program Curriculum and Scope
The Health Care IT field is an exciting, in-demand field with growing and lucrative opportunities.

HC-IT Short Certificate training program:
- ✓ Industry certifications
- ✓ Options to be multi-skill qualified for employment in four to five industries

The Healthcare Information Technician Program has two programs to select from: (a) the seven-week program; and (b) the three-month program.

(a) Healthcare Information Technician Program: Seven-week program

1. HC-IT 200: Introduction to the IT for Healthcare Environment and Technology
2. HC-IT 201: Information Technology for Healthcare Language
3. HC-IT 202: Healthcare Information Technology Mobile Devices
4. HC-IT 203: Healthcare Computer Basics
5. Registered Nurse Aide Course
6. Microsoft Word
7. PACS Training

Scope

1. HC-IT 201: Information Technology for Healthcare Language
2. HC-IT 202: Healthcare Information Technology Mobile Devices
3. HC-IT 203: Healthcare Computer Basics
4. HC-IT 200: Introduction to the IT for Healthcare Environment and Technology

Registered Nurse Aide Course
Seven hours of HIV/AIDS Trainings for Licensure

Microsoft Certification for Application Specialist Word Courses
Word 2007

Emphasizes text; teaches students how to make lists and use style, a tool that helps an author format a document. Learn how to get from one place to another in a document so that you can make changes anywhere on the page. Learn how to add text, delete text, and move text around. Learn how to utilize the basic functions of Word: type where you want to on a page, fix spelling errors, change spacing and page margins, and save your work.

PACS Training Courses
Certified PACS Associate (CPAS): This certification is achieved by passing the two exams listed below.
- CPAS-Technical: Individuals are able to demonstrate their knowledge of general technical skills.
- CPAS-Clinical: Individuals are able to demonstrate their knowledge of general clinical skills.

(b) Healthcare Information Technician Program: Three-month program

1.	HC-IT 200: Introduction to the IT for Healthcare Environment and Technology
2.	HC-IT 201: Information Technology for Healthcare Language
3.	HC-IT 202: Healthcare Information Technology Mobile Devices
4.	HC-IT 203: Healthcare Computer Basics
5.	Registered Nurse Aide Course
6.	Certified Nurse Aide
7.	Microsoft Word
8.	Microsoft Excel
9.	PACS Training

Scope

1. HC-IT 200: Introduction to the IT for Healthcare Environment and Technology
2. HC-IT 201: Information Technology for Healthcare Language
3. HC-IT 203: Healthcare Computer Basics
4. HC-IT 204: Healthcare Information Technology Implementation
5. HC-IT 234: Mobile Devices in the Healthcare Environment - Smartphones, PDAs, Medical Modalities, Laptops, and Desktops

(Option 1) Certified Nurse Aide Courses

A certificate nurse assisting program prepares students to provide daily patient care. Applicants to a certificate program in nurse assisting must receive a series of vaccinations for infectious diseases before enrolling. Vaccination is required because many certificate nurse assisting programs include a clinical experience course.

(Option 2) Registered Nurse Aide Course

Seven hours of HIV/AIDS trainings for licensure

Microsoft Certification for Application Specialist Word and Excel 2007 Courses

Word 2007

Emphasizes text; teaches students how to make lists and use style, a tool that helps an author format a document. Learn how to get from one place to another in a document so that you can make changes anywhere on the page. Learn how to add text, delete text, and move text around. Learn how to utilize the basic functions of Word: type where you want to on a page, fix spelling errors, change spacing and page margins, and save your work.

Excel 2007

Emphasizes text; teaches students how to make lists and use style, a tool that helps an author format a spreadsheet. Learn how to get from one place to another in a spreadsheet so that you can make changes anywhere within the spreadsheet. Learn how to add text, delete text, and move text around. Learn how to utilize the basic functions of Excel: type where you want to on a page, fix spelling errors, change spacing and page margins, and save your work.

PACS Training Courses
Certified PACS Associate (CPAS): This certification is achieved by passing both of the exams listed below.

- CPAS-Technical: Individuals are able to demonstrate their knowledge of general technical skills.
- CPAS-Clinical: Individuals are able to demonstrate their knowledge of general clinical skills. The course curriculum includes computer systems troubleshooting, HIPAA training, computer network troubleshooting, and UNIX system troubleshooting.

Professional Training Program

Professional Training
This course includes instructor-led training on writing business letters, learning to use Microsoft products, communication skills, understanding workflow processes, office computer understanding, and customer service understanding.

Basic Computer Skills
This course includes instructor-led training on writing letters, reports, essays, poems, and stories, as well as adding images using Microsoft Office products, office computer understanding, and customer service understanding.

Customer Service
This course includes instructor-led training on communication and listening skills, reading body language, tone and professionalism, pro-activeness and problem-solving, office computer understanding, and customer service understanding.

Transitional Skills

This course includes instructor-led training on communication and listening skills, professionalism, pro-activeness, problem-solving, resume writing, office computer understanding, and customer service understanding.

"EMR" Transitional Skills

This course includes instructor-led electronic medical records transitional skills, including training on hiring, software, medical application skills, and implementation skills, understanding the systems process, office computer understanding, and customer service understanding.

Cell/Mobile Phone Technician

This course includes instructor-led training on understanding Smartphone processes and cell/mobile phone technical environments, office computer understanding, and customer service understanding.

Microsoft Office 2007

This course includes instructor-led training on learning to use various Microsoft Office 2007 products in a business setting, office computer understanding, and customer service understanding.

Microsoft Office 2003

This course includes instructor-led training on learning to use various Microsoft Office 2003 products in a business setting, office computer understanding, and customer service understanding.

Resume Writing Course

This course includes instructor-led training on resumes and their important components, effective key word usage, office computer understanding, and customer service understanding.

Computer Skills

This advanced-level course includes instructor-led training on writing letters, reports, essays, poems, and stories, as well as adding images using Microsoft Office products, office computer understanding, and customer service understanding.

Health Care and Computers
This course includes instructor-led training on health care and computers, office computer understanding, and customer service understanding.

Software Testing
This course includes instructor-led training on software testing, office computer understanding, and customer service understanding.

New Software in the Workplace
This course includes instructor-led training on understanding and using new software in the workplace (as well as its various components), office computer understanding, and customer service understanding.

Front Office Skills
This course includes office computer understanding and customer service understanding.

The HC-IT Program

Industry Focus
Stimulus-driven positions in the medical field include Help Desk Technician, Clinical Support Staff, Data Specialist, Radiology Assistant, Radiology Office Assistant, and Certified Nurse Aide, and numerous other HC-IT positions that revolve around the entry-level, call center environment. In the field of Information Technology, students can be employed in entry-level positions such as Tech Support Specialist.

The HC-IT Program Associate of Applied Science

Prerequisites: At least three IT certifications

HC-IT Courses
- HC-IT 200: Introduction to the IT for Healthcare Environment and Technology
- HC-IT 201: Information Technology for Healthcare Language
- HC-IT 202: Health Care Information Technology Mobile Devices
- HC-IT 203: Health Care Computer Basics
- HC-IT 204 Health Care Information Technology Implementation
- HC-IT 205: Health Care Information Technology and EMR
- HC-IT 205: Health Care Information Technology Medical Applications
- HC-IT 235: IT for Healthcare Language
- HC-IT 234: Mobile Devices in the Healthcare Environment

Scope of the Overall Program

The HC-IT for Healthcare Program has three components for students, depending on their choice and background of careers in the rapidly expanding IT for health care field. The three components include AAS, One-Year Achievement Certificate, and Short-Term Certificate.

AAS-T Degree Scope
The AAS-T degree in HC-IT program is a three-career pathway degree that includes training for three IT health care industry certifications. It is a unique degree that will enable graduates to work in the medical field in hospitals, home health, radiology departments, health care call centers, and ambulatory care facilities.

In the medical field, students can be employed in entry-level positions such as Help Desk Technician, Clinical Support Staff, Data Specialist, Radiology Assistant, Radiology Office Assistant, and Certified Nurse Aide, in addition to an entry-level position in a call center environment. In the information technology field, students can be employed in entry-level positions, such as Tech Support Specialist.

Scope of HC-IT Courses

HC-IT 200: Introduction to the IT for Open Health Care Environment and Technology

HC-IT 202: Health Care Information Open Technology Mobile Devices

HC-IT 203: Health Care Computer Basics

HC-IT 204: Health Care Information Technology Implementation

HC-IT 205: Health Care Information Technology and EMR

HC-IT 206: Health Care Information Technology Medical Applications

HC-IT 234: Mobile Devices in the Health Care Environment
- Smartphones
- PDAs
- Medical Modalities
- Laptops
- Desktops

HC-IT 235: IT for Health Care Language
- Uses of medical terminology in IT for Health Care
- Workflow of the medical environment

HC-IT Certifications Study Guide Topics

- Health care
- Health care terms (HHS.gov, 2010)
- Health care and computers
- Software testing
- Cell phones
- New software in the workplace
- Business processes
- Accounts and workflow

Sample Principal Qualifications for a Health Care Information Technology Analyst / Stimulus Team Member / Implementation Experience

Business Analyst
- Coordinates with IT application analysts and other departmental analysts
- Recruits and markets training workshops, customizes standardized pre-approved brochures and formats, etc.
- Draws from feedback and makes quality improvements in workshop delivery and content
- Collects, inputs, and reports data to maintain records
- Works with hardware and a variety of secure networks across several agencies and locations

Server Support Analyst
- Implements security user accounts on new and existing servers
- Works with staff to ensure that stored data is protected by adequate access restrictions
- Conducts training on network resources
- Installs SAN network connections
- Performs functions in Server Troubleshooting/Client problems using Remote Desktop Support
- Collects, inputs, and reports data to maintain records

- Works with hardware and a variety of secure networks across several agencies and locations
- Solves problems creatively and effectively performs technical troubleshooting onsite

Program Coordinator
- Customizes and delivers pre-existing technology curricula for job seekers, including lessons that simulate work environments and work-based learning projects
- Implements secure user accounts on new and existing servers
- Defines and creates appropriate user groups within Microsoft server 2003 and/or 2008
- Performs server and active directory administration
- Works with staff to ensure that stored data is protected by adequate access restrictions
- Performs functions in server troubleshooting/client problems via remote desktop support

Systems Support Analyst/Trainer
- Documents, tracks, and monitors problems to ensure timely resolution
- Creates virtual networks to test new systems using VM Ware and Virtual PC
- Trains staff on Microsoft applications, Microsoft Office computer applications, computer repair, and Outlook applications
- Performs functions in solutions design and software implementation
- Performs troubleshooting on software applications
- Delivers clear, concise, and engaging technology training for group and individual audiences, including older youth and mature workers

Network Systems Analyst/Student/Internship
- Serves as Network Support Analyst between system users and

46

the technical support group
- Performs training on common operating systems and Microsoft Office (98, 2000, 2003, XP)
- Manipulates data via MS DOS
- Performs technical support on printers, networks, and software installations
- Performs technical support for software application issues
- Communicates clearly and effectively with customers and staff
- Uses the remote desktop method to assist and troubleshoot software issues

Computer Programmer
- Designs, develops, and implements web sites
- Troubleshoots, debugs, and implements software code
- Provides solutions for design and software implementation issues
- Creates user groups and user case workflows

Application Analyst
- Performs scanning tasks
- Conducts training on Med Manager Billing Software for surrounding hospitals
- Upgrades software using MS Excel and MS Access
- Assists with overall project management

Customer Service Rep
- Performs technical support on printers, networks, and software installations
- Performs technical support for software application issues
- Communicates clearly and effectively with customers and staff

Nursing Aide
- Explains policies and procedures to patients and refers them to the proper departments
- Communicates patients' questions, complaints, problems, and

47

concerns to appropriate staff members

Other books that might be of interest:

Health Care Information Technology
The Hardware and Software Focus:
Critical Factors for Medical Systems Implementation

<u>2nd Revision 2011</u>

ISBN-10 0615447767

ISBN-13 9780615447766

HC-IT-SC is in collaborations with various authors, educational organizations, and health care organizations for creating educational material. So please search for our material on Amazon.com or Createspace.

Health Care Information Technology Definitions

Below is a list of important definitions for health care technology professionals and those wishing to better understand and implement the provisions of HIPAA and the ARRA.

Applications Analysis – Support given to a certain application, which may entail some programming, system administration, problem analysis and diagnosis, finding the root cause of the problem, and solving the problem. Typically "applications analysis" includes supporting custom applications programmed with a variety of programming languages and using a variety of database systems, middleware systems and the like. It is a form of third-level line technical support.[7]

Authenticate – Allow access with the minimum requirement of having the user supply a username and a password.

Authorization – Allowing a user to access only categories of information allowed by permission of a supervisor or other superior.

Browser – Program used for accessing information on a network such as the World Wide Web.

Business Systems – Methodical procedures or processes, used as delivery mechanisms for providing specific goods or services to customers in a well-defined market.[8]

Cell Phone – Hand-held mobile radiotelephone for use in an area divided into small sections, each with its own short-range

---

[7]   "Application Analyst," 2010

[8]   "Business System," 2010

transmitter/receiver.[9]

Cell Technician – Carries out proper fault diagnosis to improve the quality of the cell phone, as well as carries out repairs on mobile phones to improve the phones' productivity. The main services offered by a cell phone technician are making repairs, keeping customers informed about services provided by the company (including warranties and after-sales services), and providing advice and recommendations about phones.[10]

Certified Nurse Aide/Patient Care Assistant – Person who assists individuals with health care needs (often called "patients," "clients," "service users") with activities of daily living (ADLs) and provides bedside care—including basic nursing procedures—all under the supervision of a Registered Nurse (RN) or Licensed Practical Nurse (LPN).[11]

CPT codes – Coding system for medical procedures that allows for comparability in billing, pricing, and utilization review.[12]

Confidentiality – Sensitive data must be encrypted.

Customer Service – Service provided to a paying or non-paying customer or client of any business.

Data Integrity – Data sent across the network cannot be modified by an unauthorized user or the process and/or means of transportation.

Digital Healthcare Environment – A form of Electronic Health Recording. A DHE is a more secure environment which demands both advanced encryption and authentication processes for the users, thereby securing client information.

---

[9]   "Cell Phone," 2010
[10]   Muchira, 2010
[11]   "Certified Nursing Assistant," 2010
[12]   "CPT Codes," 2009

EHR (Electronic Health Record) – The aggregate electronic record of health-related information on an individual that is created and gathered cumulatively across more than one health care organization and is managed and used by licensed clinicians and staff involved in the individual's health and care.[13]

EMR (Electronic Medical Record) – The electronic record of health-related information on an individual that is created, gathered, managed, and used by licensed clinicians and staff from a single organization who are involved in the individual's health and care.[14]

Hardware – All-inclusive term for the physical parts of a computer, as distinguished from the data it has or operates on.[15]

HCPC Codes (Healthcare Common Procedure Coding) – System of letter and number codes designated to procedures, supplies, medications, and equipment that are used for pricing and billing.[16]

Healthcare Information Management – Management of all patient data within a health care facility.

Healthcare Information Technology – Support and/or management of the hardware and software in a health care facility.[17]

Health Information Privacy – The Office of Civil Rights enforces each of the following: the HIPAA Privacy Rule, which protects the privacy of individually identifiable health information; the HIPAA Security Rule, which sets national standards for the security of electronic protected health information; and the confidentiality provisions of the Patient Safety Rule, which protects identifiable

---

[13]   Neal, 2008
[14]   Ibid
[15]   "Computer Hardware Definition," 2010
[16]   "Glossary of Definitions," 2007
[17]   "Health Information Careers: Glossary of Terms," 2010

information from being used to analyze patient safety events and improves patient safety.[18]

Hearing Aids – Electro-acoustic devices which usually fit in or behind the wearer's ears and are designed to increase and adjust sound for the wearer.[19]

HIPAA – The Health Insurance Portability and Accountability Act (HIPAA) was enacted by the U.S. Congress in 1996. It was originally sponsored by Sen. Edward Kennedy (D-Mass.) and Sen. Nancy Kassebaum (R-Kan.). According to the Centers for Medicare and Medicaid Services (CMS) website, Title I of HIPAA protects health insurance coverage for workers and their families when they change or lose their jobs. Title II of HIPAA, known as the Administrative Simplification (AS) provisions, requires the establishment of national standards for electronic healthcare transactions and national identifiers for providers, health insurance plans, and employers.[20]

Home Healthcare Aide – Trained and certified healthcare worker who provides assistance to a patient in the home with personal care (such as hygiene and exercise) and light household duties (such as meal preparation) and who monitors the patient's condition.[21]

IT/Information Technology – Anything related to computing technology, such as networking, hardware, software, the Internet, or the people who work with these technologies

Medical Application – Any computer software that is used in a health-care organization, and can include software that connects to medical devices such as hearing aids, medical imaging systems, remote patient monitoring and diagnostics, and medical alarm applications.

---

[18] "Understanding Health Information Privacy," 2010
[19] "Hearing Aid," 2010
[20] "Health Insurance Portability and Accountability Act," 2010
[21] "Home health aide" 2010

Medical Records – Confidential documents that contain detailed and comprehensive information on an individual and the care and experience related to that person.

Medical Software Systems – Fully integrated system that allows full access to scheduling, transcription and document management for any healthcare office.

Medical Financial Applications Specialist – Analyzes and defines financial management and project systems functions and business processes and user needs; also analyzes and evaluates existing business functions and processes related to general accounting, accounts receivable/payable, inventory, budget, and procurement activities.[22]

Patient Care – Services rendered by members of the health profession and non-professionals under their supervision for the benefit of the patient.

Project Management – Management of Information Technology projects. Planning and execution of any project from start to finish.

Proxy – Intermediary (that is, a middle-man or go-between) for requests between a workstation and another server. The proxy acts as a filter for information, delivering only what was within the request description.

Requirements – Definition for the software based on functionality.

Role – Description of what any system or program is designed to do

Server – Computer system or application program that provides services to multiple computers and users.

Software – Programs and data held in the storage of a computer used to direct the operation of a computer, as well as any documentation that

---

[22] "Article Search Results for Medical Cash Applications Specialist," 2010

provides instructions on how to use those programs.[23]

Super User – On many computer operating systems, the super user, or root, is a special user account used for system administration.[24]

---

[23]   "Software Definition," 2010
[24]   "Superuser," 2010

Affiliates

The author wishes to thank the Health Care Information Technology Service Center (HC-IT-SC) and the Information Technology Center (ITC) for their affiliation with this project and for their generous support.

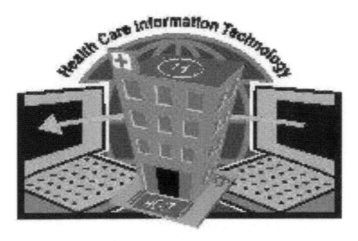

Feedback

The book you hold in your hands is part of a series intended to give professionals the most useful and up-to-date information necessary to ensure satisfactory outcomes in the field of Healthcare IT. However, our ability to provide this information is greatly shaped by the invaluable feedback of our readers.

We welcome your suggestions, comments, and recommendations for future books in this series, and your input allows us to better serve your specific needs as we continue to publish additional information. We would be honored if you'd share with us what you'd like to see!

Please send all comments and suggestions to:

HC-IT-SC
Re: Book Feedback
P.O. Box 3388
Federal Way, WA 98063

References

1. "Computer Networks: Chapter 12 - The Network Development Life Cycle." *csc.colstate.edu*. Oct. 2010. (csc.colstate.edu/summers/notes/cs457/chapt12.htm)

2. "Health Information Technology." *Wikipedia*. October 2010. Wikipedia. 13 Oct. 2010. http://en.wikipedia.org/wiki/Health_information_technology# Concepts_and_Definitions

3. "Article Search Results for Medical Cash Applications Specialist." *eHow*. 18 Oct. 2010. http://www.ehow.com/search.aspx?s= medical+cash+applications+specialist&Options=0

4. Neal, Houston. "EHR vs. EMR – What's the Difference?" *Softwareadvice.com*. November 2008. 13 Oct. 2010. http://www.softwareadvice.com/articles/medical/ehr-vs-emr-whats-the-difference/

5. "Existing Medical Record Number (MRN) based identification." *National Committee on Vital and Health Statistics*. October 2010. 14 Oct. 2010. http://www.ncvhs.hhs.gov/app7-8.htm

6. "The History of the Computer." *MerchantOs*. Oct. 2010. 13 Oct. 2010, http://www.merchantos.com/articles/informational/the-history-of-the-computer/

7. "Application Analyst." *Wikipedia*. 12 Oct. 2010. 18 Oct. 2010. http://en.wikipedia.org/wiki/Application_analyst

8. "Business System." *Business Dictionary.com*. 18 Oct. 2010. http://www.businessdictionary.com/definition/business-system.html

9. "Cell Phone." The Free Dictionary." 18 Oct. 2010. http://www.thefreedictionary.com/cellphone

10. Muchira, Martin. "Cellphone Technician Job Description." *eHow*. 12 July 2010. 18 October 2010. http://www.ehow.com/about_6722228_cell-phone-technician-job-description.html

11. "Certified Nursing Assistant." *Wikipedia.* 18 Oct. 2010.
http://en.wikipedia.org/wiki/Certified_nursing_assistant

12. "CPT Codes." *Medical-dictionary.thefreedictionary.com.* 18
October 2010.
http://www.medical-
dictionary.thefreedictionary.com/CPT+codes

13. Neal, Houston. "EHR vs. EMR – What's the Difference?"
Softwareadvice.com. November 2008. 13 Oct. 2010.
http://www.softwareadvice.com/articles/medical/ehr-vs-emr-
whats-the-difference/

14. Neal, Houston. "EHR vs. EMR – What's the Difference?"
Softwareadvice.com. November 2008. 13 Oct. 2010.
http://www.softwareadvice.com/articles/medical/ehr-vs-emr-
whats-the-difference/

15. "Computer Hardware Definition." *Open Projects.* 18 Oct. 2010.
http://www.openprojects.org/hardware-definition.htm

16. "Glossary of Definitions." *Cahaba Government Benefits
Administrators, LLC.* 24 May 2007. 18 October 2010.
http://www.cahabagba.com/glossary/definitions/content1n9.htm
l

17. "Health Information Careers: Glossary of Terms." *Ahima.*18
Oct. 2010.
http://hicareers.com/Health_Information_101/glossary.aspx

18. "Understanding Health Information Privacy." *U.S. Department
of Health and Human Services.* 12 June 2010.
http://www.hhs.gov/ocr/privacy/hipaa/understanding/index.html

19. "Hearing Aid." *Wikipedia.* 18 October 2010.
http://en.wikipedia.org/wiki/Hearing_aid

20. "Health Insurance Portability and Accountability Act."
Wikipedia. 18 Oct. 2010.
http://en.wikipedia.org/wiki/Health_Insurance_Portability_and_
Accountability_Act

21. "Home health aide." *Dictionary.com.* 18 Oct. 2010.
http://dictionary.reference.com/browse/home+health+aide

22. "Article Search Results for Medical Cash Applications
Specialist." *eHow.* 18 Oct. 2010.
http://www.ehow.com/search.aspx?s=

medical+cash+applications+specialist&Options=0
23. "Software Definition." *WordIQ.com*. 18 Oct. 2010.
   http://www.wordiq.com/definition/Software
24. "Superuser." *Wikipedia*. 19 Oct. 2010
   http://en.wikipedia.org/wiki/Superuser

Further Reading

"Accounting Terms – Glossary of Accounting Terms and Definitions."
Buzzle. 12 June 2010.
http://www.buzzle.com/articles/accounting-terms-glossary-of-
accounting-terms-and-definitions.html

"Biba Model." *Wikipedia*. 2 December 2009. 12 June 2010.
http://en.wikipedia.org/wiki/Biba_model

"Business Process Modeling." *Businessballs.com*. 14 July 2010.
http://www.businessballs.com/business-process-
modelling.htm#BPMdefinition

"Health Information Management." *The Free Dictionary*. Farlex. 13
Oct. 2010.
http://encyclopedia.thefreedictionary.com/health+information+manage
ment

"Health Information Manager." *Healthposts.com.au*. 13 Oct. 2010.
http://www.healthposts.com.au/job/health-information-
manager_1000.htm

"Health Information Management." *Wikipedia*. 13 Oct. 2010.
http://en.wikipedia.org/wiki/Health_information_management

"ICD-10 Compliance." *TM Floyd & Company: Building Better
Solutions*. 18 Oct. 2010.

http://www.icd-10compliance.com/factors.asp

"Micro Instrumentation and Telemetry System." *Wikipedia*. 18 Oct.
2010.
http://en.wikipedia.org/wiki/Micro_Instrumentation_and_Telemetry_Sy
stems

"PACS Administrators Registry and Certification Association." *PACS
Admin*. 12 June 2010.
http://www.pacsadmin.org/

Pan, Jiantao. "Software Testing". *Carnegie Melon University*. 12 June
2010. http://www.ece.cmu.edu/~koopman/des_s99/sw_testing/
#concepts

"ProcessMaker is your Open Source BPM Software Solution."
ProcessMaker. May 2010. 12 June 2010.
http://www.processmaker.com/

Straube, Diana M. "HPCPS Codes: Frequently Asked Questions."
Neighborhood Legal Services. November 2008. 12 June 2010
http://www.nls.org/av/FAQ%27s%20HCPCS.pdf

Tran, Eushiuan. "Verification/Validation/Certification." *Carnegie
Melon University*. 1999. 14 June 2010.
http://www.ece.cmu.edu/~koopman/des_s99/verification/index. html

"WikiAnswers." *Answers.com*. 2010. 12 June 2010.
http://wiki.answers.com/Q/Where_in_North_America_is_area_
code_973.

9611297R0003

Made in the USA
Charleston, SC
28 September 2011